The 80-20 Diet

I0436296

MY BLOG   **FREE BOOKS**   **OUR AUDIOS**   **OUR MOVIE**

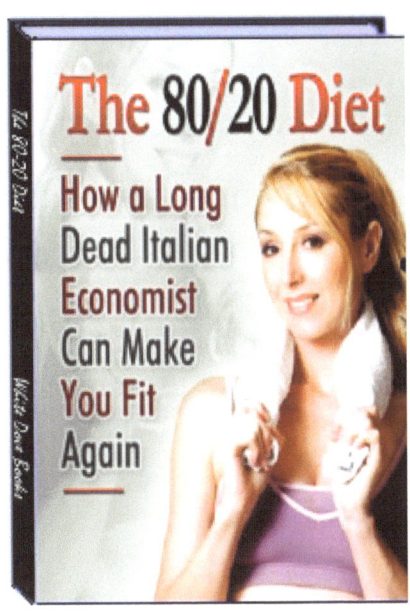

Statement of Rights

You may sell this book for profit or you may give it away or use it as a bonus. You may **NOT** change it in any way.

Copyright Message

PLR Obtained by White Dove Books 2008

http://www.whitedovebooks.co.uk

Disclaimer

Reasonable care has been taken to ensure that the information presented in this book is accurate. However, the reader should understand that the information provided does not constitute legal, medical or professional advice of <u>any</u> kind.

No Liability: this product is supplied "as is" and without warranties. <u>All</u> warranties, express or implied, are hereby disclaimed.

Use of this product constitutes acceptance of the "No Liability" policy. If you do not agree with this policy, you are not permitted to use or distribute this product.

White Dove Books, its employees, associates, distributors, agents and affiliates shall not be liable for any losses or damages whatsoever (including, without limitation, consequential loss or damage) directly or indirectly arising from the use of this product.

Contents

Introduction

We all want to stay fit. We all want a healthy body. We all want to feel proud of ourselves when someone compliments us about our good shape. We all want to lose our extra fat, bring down our weight and do everything that we wanted to do for years – LOOK GOOD.

There are gazillion methods of weight loss that are being taught but some way or the other, nothing seems to work out for some people. If you're anything like me, you've probably tried all kinds of exercises like aerobics, strength training etc. and dieting with all types of plans that literally make you feel like you are STARVING to death but still don't help you lose weight.

What's wrong with those exercises and diet plans? What are we doing wrong here? The problem is that we are putting in the effort, but we are not directing it at the right place.

Vilfredo Pareto was a French-Italian sociologist, economist and philosopher who was born on July 15, 1848. He is famous for describing an interesting principle which you might have heard about. It is called the Pareto Principle and it states that:

80% of your results come from 20% of your efforts

He had originally noticed how 80% of the income in Italy went to just 20% of the population; but his principle has been found to have application in many other fields as well.

If you apply this principle to weight loss, it necessitates doing only those things which will give you the BEST results. So, you have to do only those 20% exercises which give you 80% of all your results. You have to cut down on that 20% of food that results in 80% of your fat.

Once you do that, it will become very easy to lose weight.

In this ebook, I am going to share with you **The 80/20 Diet** – my personal system that can help you lose 20 pounds in just 30 days!

Having tried all the diet and exercise plans on the market and seeing them fail, I was really de-motivated. I didn't like the way I looked with all the fat on my body but I felt I really couldn't help it either. I tried everything from cardio exercises to low cabbage-soup diets but nothing worked for me. I even took up fasting for a week to see if it would help, but all to no avail.

That was probably the most frustrating time of my life. But then, I hate being helpless. I just couldn't sit there and see myself get even fatter. I decided that this had to change; and so I started on my quest to finding the perfect system for weight loss. I looked on the Internet, I consulted doctors and read magazines. I did everything within my power to find help for myself.

After a lot of reseach, I realized that it's not just a single plan or exercise that would help me. Instead, it's a whole combination of things that would work together to help me lose weight. In the 80/20 Diet, I bring to you the same techniques that I used to lose all my fat and return to a perfectly normal weight myself.

Let's begin…

Chapter 1:

Debunking the Myths

Before I introduce you to the system, it is important to debunk some old myths about weight loss as well as take a critical look at the various diet and exercise plans out there which don't work as intended.

First, let's see why people gain weight in the first place:

a. Overeating

"Eating more than you can burn" not surprisingly, is the main reason for weight gain. Our busy lives provide us with too little time to spend on eating healthily. So we pick up that packet of tortilla chips or order a Big Mac while on our way to the office. The problem is that these things contain a lot of calories and fat which, again thanks to our busy schedule, will remain unburned since we tend to exercise so little.

b. Lack of Exercise

As I mentioned above, a total lack of exercise in your life will surely lead to weight gain. If you are physically inactive in your daily life and are mainly doing your work whilst seated (as is the case in most modern office work) you are more likely to gain weight – and fast too!

c. Genetic Reasons

Some people may gain weight simply due to their genes. If their parents (or one of the parents) are obese, the child may grow to be obese as well.

d. Stress & Depression

Believe it or not, stress and depression can result in weight gain too. This is simply because people often resort to overeating as a response to emotional pressures like stress and depression and hence end up gaining weight. This is sometimes called 'Emotional Eating'.

e. Pregnancy

Pregnant women who have just delivered a baby will usually notice an increase in their weight of perhaps somewhere around an additional 4 to 6 pounds.

f. Quitting Smoking

When a heavy smoker quits smoking altogether, he/she may notice a weight gain of 5 to 10 pounds. This is because smoking reduces appetite (because of the nicotine in cigarettes) and also increases the metabolic rate (although slightly) so that the body burns more calories. When you quit smoking, your eating may increase while your metabolism goes down - leading to unwanted weight gain.

There are a number of other reasons why one may gain weight but these are the major ones. The challenges of modern life, stress, depression, lack of exercise, physical inactivity and wrong choices of food are only some reasons why people gain weight. And being over weight is not good because it increases the chances of cardiovascular diseases, diabetes, digestive system problems, low immunity towards diseases and even skin and eye diseases.

Hence, it becomes necessary to eat healthily, live healthily and exercise properly for our own benefit.

Chapter 2:

What to Eat and How

In this chapter, I will tell you what food items you must include in your diet and which ones you must reduce or, better still, completely eliminate. In identifying these items, we will be making great use of the 80/20 rule we have already discussed.

Now, the first thing you must understand is that it's vital for your body to fulfill its daily nutrient requirements. Hence, although you might decide to cut down on a few food items, you must absolutely make sure that you give your body its desired nutrition.

Let's use the 80/20 rule and decide to eliminate that 20% food from your overall diet that will help in 80% reduction of your weight.

OK now let this sink-in: if you want a healthy body, you just need to concentrate on reducing or completely eliminating the following items from your diet …

The 20% of foods that are 80% responsible for your weight problems are …

- **Flour**
- **Sugar**
- **Salt**
- **Alcohol**

That's not complicated is it? It is also not a lot to remember. But this is powerful because if you can just work on cutting-down or eliminating these foods from your diet, you will have no problems with weight at all.

Foods that contain added sugar and refined flour, quite simply, are nutrient-poor. Foods that contain whole grains, fruits, vegetables and legumes are rich in vitamins, minerals and fibre (fiber). So avoid foods containing these things - especially cakes, pastries, biscuits etc – which contain both!

Salt itself does not cause you to gain or lose fat because salt has no calories. However, a diet that is high in salt will likely affect both your blood pressure and your weight.

Why? Because high levels of salt in the modern diet usually come from processed foods which are also usually high in calories. So stick to a low-salt diet, because it will most probably consist of lower calorie, healthier foods.

Now then – alcohol! A friend of mine, who was clinically obese, completely solved his weight problem just by – guess what? Simply by giving up alcohol!

Here's something that will probably surprise you: what is usually referred to as a *beer-belly* is NOT caused by excess alcohol calories being stored as fat! It turns out that less than five percent of the alcohol calories we consume are turned into fat. The main effect of drinking alcohol is a reduction in the amount of fat our bodies burn-off as energy.

So we need to work on reducing or eliminating this stuff from your diet! Now I understand that these items may be part of your daily diet and you can't even imaging doing without them. The trick is not to cut down or eliminate them in one go, but instead proceed slowly.

So, now let the message of this book sink in. There are just those 4 food groups to remember. That's the 80/20 law! You will probably not need to reduce **all** of them; and you do not need to completely eliminate – just cut-down! OK, that said, let's consider how to do it.

How to Cut-Down - Let's Consider Sugar as an Example

If you've been eating sugar (in any of its forms) since childhood, it's nearly impossible to stop eating it - *tomorrow*!

What you have to do is cut down your daily sugar intake by small amounts. For example, if you take a total of 5 cups of sugary drinks per day (tea, coffee, sodas etc), you could begin by moving that total down to, say 4 or even 3 cups. That way, you won't feel the 'pain' of having to do without it and still be able to control yourself. After a couple of weeks, you can cut it down to just 2 cups.

Better still, try to learn to take those drinks without sugar or perhaps try replacing them (or some of them) with herbal drinks that do not contain sugar. Just cut-down; you don't need to cut them out completely. Really? Yes!

It's easy. Isn't it?

The goal is to make small changes that will bring in huge results – that's the 80/20 principle at work - and that's how you have to proceed. We're not cutting out everything. Rather, we're cutting-out, or down, on only that small number of items that are responsible for generating a lot of fat in the body - or don't give it a chance to burn body fat.

But your body is probably quite used to taking in a lot of those items each week. So how do you teach it to live without them in such a short period of time? Well, here's what I suggest: **eat anything you want every 5th day**! Yes I really did say that – and I think I'll say it again for effect because that's the power of the Pareto Diet: **eat anything you want every 5th day**!

Every 5th day, I am suggesting that you eat ANYTHING you want! You could eat chocolate or drink coffee or maybe beer or eat cakes or pasta – just about anything. This will fulfill your body's need to eat what it likes while still keeping your weight under control.

This approach will shake-up your body and keep you on-track to losing that excess weight even though you're eating pretty-much whatever you like on that one day. Again this is the 80/20 law coming into play – you will be eating healthily for 80% of the time; and allowing yourself 20% of the time (1 day in every 5) to have a break from your regime.

This will keep you interested in this lifestyle change permanently. If you have a special occasion coming up - that means you will be eating and/or drinking some of the items we listed - that's ok, just don't do it more than once in every 5 day period.

That's also why eating out should be avoided – for 80% of the time anyway! Quite simply, food at many restaurants is often not as healthy as home made food; often containing because high-salt, processed ingredients. And in addition, you may decide to have a dessert course (even if you are not hungry) which is full of flour and sugar. And furthermore, you will probably consume some alcohol too! This, of course will result in increasing the fat in your body.

Four days out of every five, try hard to reduce just those four things and you will find that Pareto's Principle will work for you. On those four days, make eating healthy food your top priority in your diet. You don't need to starve yourself when you go on a diet. All you have to do is cut-down on just the right food items so that you get the best results in the shortest amount of time.

Chapter 3:

How to Exercise for Weight Loss

OK, so we now know what to eat, what not to eat and how frequently, to do it. What I now want to share with you is how you can get even quicker results by combining exercise. In this chapter, I will share with you the proper exercise routines that will go along with your new diet plan.

Exercise is as important for your body as is a healthy and balanced diet. I can't emphasize it enough – exercise is a fantastic accelerator for losing weight and keeping your body healthy.

But as with food, we're going to apply the Pareto principle to exercising as well. See, there is exercise and then there is good exercise. Good exercise is that exercise that really benefits your body. By applying the 80/20 rule to exercising, you will only need to do that 20% of exercise that gives you highest amount of results - that sounds good doesn't it?

Are you ready? Then let's begin.

It does not matter too-much exactly what type of physical exercise you perform – playing sport, gardening, performing house-hold tasks – absolutely *all* forms of exercise are beneficial to a certain extent.

However, Pareto's Principle tells us that 20% of the exercise we engage in will result in 80% of the benefit – and that kind of exercise is – *aerobic* exercise. That's the kind of exercise that raises the heart-rate a little.

In addition to weight-loss benefits, aerobic exercise may decrease the risk of CAD (coronary artery disease) and related *comobidites*. That's an interesting medical word isn't it? It means: the effect of all other diseases an individual patient might have other than the primary disease.

You should aim to exercise two or three times per week; doing sessions of 20 to 30 minutes minimum of aerobic exercise. This really is very little time to invest to reap the associated positive health benefits.

Easy Ways of Taking Aerobic Exercise

- Walking (at a reasonable pace)
- Jogging

- Riding a Bike
- Dancing
- Swimming

The best piece of advice you can get here is this – *listen carefully* – find something that you really enjoy, that is also *aerobic* by nature. If you enjoy doing it, you will be much more likely to continue and get it into your lifestyle; and that should be your intention. Conversely, if you choose to do something you don't enjoy, it will become a chore; and eventually, you will give it up.

One thing you must keep in mind is that you should never OVER-EXERCISE. No exercise is better than over-exercise! There is no need to overdo it. Since you'll be changing your diet, it will itself contribute to losing weight fast. Combine this with only as much exercise that you need – that's Pareto's Principle!

Remember -you are not training to be an athlete; you are simply asking your body to do a little extra work to enjoy the positive health benefits that will ensue. You are not here to exhaust yourself. Exercise is meant to rejuvenate your body (and mind) and keep you healthy and fit – not tired and unhealthy.

The end result is that your body burns a higher amount of calories making it a very efficient, fat-burning, healthy and fit 'machine'.

Chapter 4:

Diet Supplements

By now you know what diet you have to follow and what kind of exercise routine you should follow. In this chapter, I want to share with you some the diet supplements you might like to consider while you're losing weight.

Let's firstly consider vitamin tablets. Now, you will need to make your own mind up about this issue, but personally I don't recommend them. Here's why: in order for you to benefit from vitamins, they must be accompanied by the correct nutrients. For example, you need iron to absorb vitamin C; that's why you often do find iron added to vitamin C tablets.

There are many such similar vitamin/nutrient dependencies. However – every naturally occurring vitamin is packaged by mother-nature, within the natural foodstuff itself, with the necessary minerals and nutrients the body needs in order to use them!

Here's a bit of general advice on the subject of vitamins:

1. ALWAYS consult your doctor before you opt to take anything. This is true not only for multivitamins but most everything that's available at the medical store.

2. If you decide to take them, capsules, liquids or powders are generally better than pills because they are usually easier to breakdown and absorb for your body.

3. Again, if you do elect to take multivitamins, it's advisable to take them with food. This makes it a bit easier for your body to absorb them.

4. Finally, avoid multivitamins that contain too much iron. Excessive iron is known to cause problems (sometimes severely so). It may generate free radicals in your body which is NOT good.

Stay on the safer side with multivitamins by consulting your doctor about them before you think of taking any of them.

Here is a natural supplement you should consider …

According to Pareto, there will be some natural high-leverage supplements responsible for the 80% benefit! One such supplement is fish oil.

Fish oil has long been associated with weight loss and dieting. Fish oil is made from the tissues of oily fish. The reason why it is recommended as part of a healthy diet is due to the omega-3 fatty acid that it contains. This includes eicosapentaenoic acid (EPA) and docosahexaenoic acid (DHA).

Fish oil helps keep your cholesterol levels under control. So, if you're overweight or obese, it can help you stay healthy and fit while you're losing weight. It is also good for the overall health of your body.

You can opt for fish oil supplements which are available as tablets, capsules and liquids. Fish oil is not directly helpful in weight loss but it does help in the proper functioning of many body parts which surely assists you in your weight loss efforts.

So now you know about my 80/20 Diet Plan that will help you lose all the weight you want in a very short time. Now, the most important thing that will make the difference and decide if this plan works out for you or not is simply TAKING ACTION! I hope that you are use the information in this ebook to make a difference in your life – starting NOW!

Here's to a Healthier & Slimmer **You**!

The Most <u>Amazing Benefits</u> in Your Very First Week ...

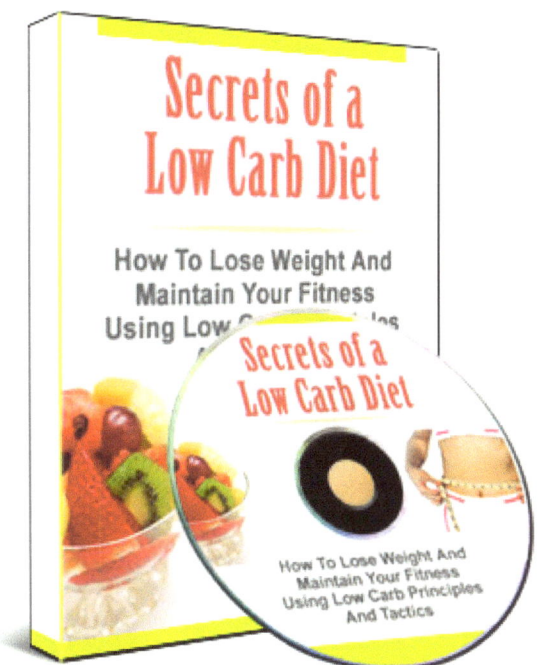

With our program **you** can realize massive improvements within a very short time.

Did you know **you** can literally transform your life and experience truly remarkable health benefits within just **<u>1 week</u>**?

In fact, here are just a few of the simply **amazing benefits** you will be experiencing by the end of your very first week ...

⭐**Immediate weight loss** of up to **<u>11 pounds</u>** in your **very first week.**

⭐**Permanent weight loss** - steadily lose weight **<u>every week</u>** to achieve permanent weight loss!

⭐**Decreased fatigue** - feel healthier, fitter, full of energy and much more alive.

⭐**Improved self-esteem** as you lose weight and feel better about the body you live in.

⭐**Increased levels of HDL** in your body - which research suggests may protect against cardiovascular disease.

⭐**Increased muscle mass** which can boost your metabolism and result in ongoing weight loss.

<u>Click Here</u> for More Details ...

The 7 Keys to Success
by Will Edwards

Another FREE Gift from White Dove Books!

The 7 Keys to Success began as a Movie at the White Dove Books site. We then made it into an eCourse for our subscribers. Now finally, it is available as a <u>FREE</u> eBook.

This book contains an important message. I hope you will get your copy and work with us to change the world.

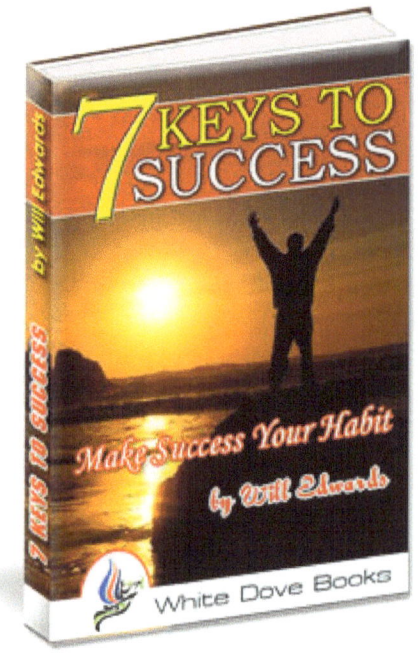

- ☑ **Commitment**

- ☑ **An Open Mind**

- ☑ **Persistence**

- ☑ **Flexibility**

- ☑ **Faith**

- ☑ **Thankfulness**

- ☑ **Passion**

☑ **INCLUDED** – You may give away this book as a free gift to your friends. You may use it as a free bonus. It may NOT be sold. You can help us to make a real difference by getting this important message to the people of the world.

<u>Click Here</u> for More Details ...

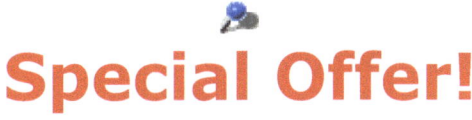

Special Offer!

COMLETE SERIES

Included in this Fabulous Package ...

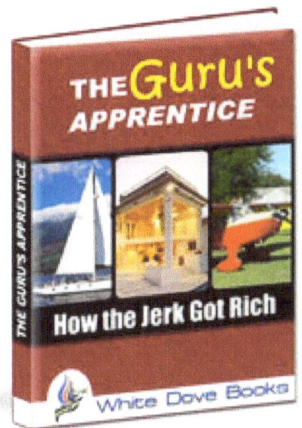

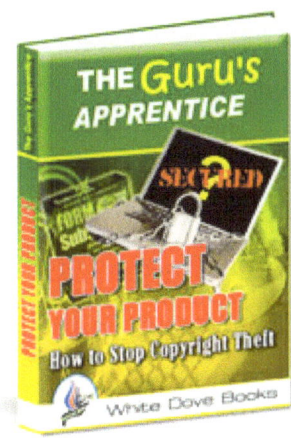

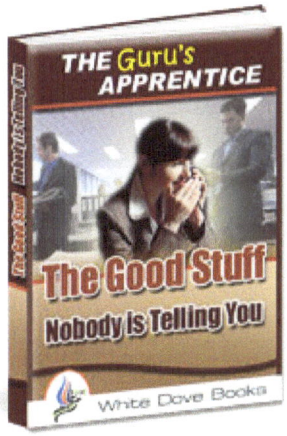

How the Rich Jerk Made Use of Advanced Subliminal Techniques

☑ Full Product
☑ Sales Page
☑ Professional Graphics
☑ Master Resale Rights

Legitimately Register Copyright without Paying Any Registration Fees

☑ Full Product
☑ Sales Page
☑ Professional Graphics
☑ Master Resale Rights

The Top 10 Secrets I am Using Right Now to Profit from the Internet

☑ Full Product
☑ Sales Page
☑ Professional Graphics
☑ Master Resale Rights

CLICK HERE FOR A VERY SPECIAL OFFER

About White Dove Books

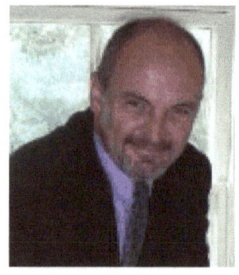

Will Edwards is the founder of White Dove Books - the internet's leading website for Self Improvement and Personal Development. A graduate of the University of Birmingham, he develops and teaches Personal Development workshops and is a published author.

Within its first three years, White Dove Books was recognised as one of the internet's leading sites for self help and personal development; breaking into the top 100,000 sites on the internet at the end of 2005.

The INSPIRATION newsletter was started in 2005 as a way of providing helpful information including tips, articles and free inspirational eBooks to our visitors.

Today White Dove Books works in partnership with many authors and on-line publishers of inspirational material to provide a quality on-line service that serves thousands of people in many countries across the world.

Our mission is to help people to develop their own unique talents, abilities and passion in order that they may lead more meaningful, joyful and fulfilled lives.

www.ingramcontent.com/pod-product-compliance
Lightning Source LLC
Chambersburg PA
CBHW060815290526
45792CB00005BB/1668